The Eye Health Cookbook

From Kitchen To Optimal Vision

Shauve Rivk

Table of Contents

Introduction

Join us as we explore the scientific process of taste chemistry and how it can convert your meal into a visual feast. The items that follow are more like a symphony of colors, sensations, and nourishment, precisely ordered to fit your eyes' delicate demands.

Every meal is a brushstroke on the canvas of your well-being, a dedication to flavor and health. Vitamins, minerals, and antioxidants are the secret heroes of our blinks and gazes, and in these chapters, we'll learn how they're related to eye health via diet.

You will learn to enjoy nature's rich palette as we deliver breakfasts to start your day, lunches to brighten your lunchtime, and nights to build to a climax of sustenance. This cookbook offers delicious dishes, but it also acts as a manifesto for a lifestyle that values and protects your eyes.

Every page gets you closer to a world in which your eyes not only see but flourish, with food that maintains your sharp eyesight and delightful pleasures that please your senses guilt-free. Join this voyage with a love for education and an open heart.

As you flip through the pages, delight in the tastes and scents, and you'll be transported to a world where each bite contributes to enhanced eyesight. Allow the visual feast to begin as you embark on your gastronomical trip.

Chapter 1: Foundations of Eye-Friendly Nutrition

Building Blocks for Healthy Vision

Vitamin A is at the forefront of ocular nutrition, and it is crucial for maintaining corneal clarity. Vitamin A, which is plentiful in vivid foods such as carrots and kale, ensures that our visual canvas stays clean.

An emerging study stresses its value in reducing night blindness and boosting general eye health. Vitamins C and E create an antioxidant alliance that protects against oxidative damage. These vitamins, which may be found in citrus fruits, berries, nuts, and seeds, serve to protect the eyes by neutralizing free radicals and may lower the occurrence of age-related illnesses.

Recent studies emphasize their role in sustaining visual acuity and retinal health. Zinc and selenium play essential roles in the design of ocular resilience. These minerals, which may be found in nuts, seeds, and whole grains, aid in building ocular tissues.

A recent study has revealed their importance in lowering the occurrence of visual impairment and age-related degenerative disorders, establishing them as key building blocks.

Omega-3 fatty acids, notably docosahexaenoic acid (DHA) and eicosapentaenoic acid (EPA), are necessary for retinal health. These fatty acids, which are plentiful in fatty fish, flaxseeds, and walnuts, aid in maintaining retinal function and may lessen the development of age-related macular degeneration.

Contemporary research adds to their narrative, stressing its cardiovascular and anti-inflammatory properties. Beyond diet, the building blocks of excellent vision include lifestyle behaviors, with protective eyewear taking center stage.

UV protection, anti-glare coatings, and blue light filters all aid in protecting our eyes from possible injury, maintaining visual acuity, and minimizing the occurrence of disorders such as cataracts.

Regular eye examinations serve as the architectural blueprints for ocular health. Comprehensive examinations not only uncover refractive issues, but they also show early symptoms of prospective eye disorders. Timely intervention becomes a cornerstone for maintaining healthy eyesight throughout life.

Vitamins and Minerals Essential for Eye Health

1. Vitamin A functions as a visual defender, protecting the purity of our corneas and giving good low-light vision. Vitamin A is plentiful in bright foods such as carrots and leafy greens, and it remains an essential component of the ocular arsenal. A recent study shows its usefulness in reducing night blindness and preserving general eye health.

2. Vitamin C, as the ocular sentinel, takes center stage, providing antioxidant defense against oxidative stress. Vitamin C, which is prevalent in citrus fruits, strawberries, and bell peppers, operates as a vital defender, neutralizing free radicals and maybe minimizing the formation of cataracts and other age-related illnesses.

3. Vitamin E, serves as a cellular defender, generating a cocoon surrounding our ocular cells. Nuts, seeds, and spinach serve as the stage for its performance. In the present debate, vitamin E's relevance goes beyond antioxidant characteristics, addressing cellular integrity and minimizing the effect of oxidative stress on eye health.

4. Zinc, an often-overlooked mineral, emerges as the architect of ocular resilience. Zinc is plentiful in seeds, nuts, and whole grains and helps to preserve the structural integrity of ocular tissues.

   A recent investigation established its importance in minimizing the incidence of visual impairment and age-related degenerative disorders, establishing it as a crucial mineral for eye health.

5. Selenium, completes the ensemble by serving as a cellular defender, safeguarding our ocular cells from oxidative stress. Selenium, which may be found in seafood, almonds, and whole grains, is

becoming increasingly recognized for its role in ocular health.

Recent discoveries underline its usefulness in the prevention of age-related illnesses and the general preservation of visual health.

Antioxidants and Their Role in Protecting the Eyes

1. **Reactive oxygen species (ROS):** The ocular battlefield is afflicted by reactive oxygen species (ROS), which are created by external sources such as UV radiation, pollution, and digital displays. These volatile molecules represent a persistent danger to the delicate structures of the eyes, generating oxidative stress and possibly harming ocular tissues.

2. **Antioxidants:** operate as attentive guards, capable of eliminating free radicals. These chemicals, available in a broad variety of foods, function as molecular firemen, halting the destructive chain events launched by ROS and

reducing the cellular damage caused to ocular tissues.

3. **Lutein and zeaxanthin:** important carotenoids present in leafy greens and bright vegetables, emerge as macular maestros. These antioxidants, which are concentrated in the macula, the center region of the retina, operate as a protective barrier against the detrimental effects of high-energy light waves, preventing age-related macular degeneration (AMD) and maintaining good central vision.

4. **Vitamin C:** is citrus's major defense against oxidative damage. This antioxidant powerhouse, which may be found in citrus fruits, strawberries, and bell peppers, plays a crucial role in ocular defense. Recent studies have proven its importance in lowering the development of cataracts and delaying the advancement of AMD, establishing it as a crucial vitamin for eye health.

5. **Vitamin E:** functions as the defender of cell integrity. Nuts, seeds, and spinach serve as stages for its performances. In the ocular story,

Vitamin E not only functions as an antioxidant but also plays a crucial role in maintaining the delicate balance of ocular cells, guarding against oxidative stress, and supporting long-term eye health.

6. **Vitamin A:** Carrots, sweet potatoes, and kale contain beta-carotene, a precursor of Vitamin A, which creates a protective covering. Beyond its antioxidant impact, beta-carotene transforms into Vitamin A in the body, strengthening the cornea and enhancing the capacity to differentiate shapes and details.

Omega-3 Fatty Acids for Retinal Health

The retina, a complex neuronal tissue lining the back of the eye, is crucial in the conversion of light into visual information. For maximum performance, the retina's delicate components, notably photoreceptor cells, require a symphony of nutrients.

The omega-3 protagonists, DHA and EPA, have proven to be retinal health defenders. These fatty acids are plentiful in fatty fish such as salmon, mackerel, and trout, and they serve to maintain the structural integrity of photoreceptor cells.

A recent study stresses their significance in sustaining visual function and minimizing the risk of age-related macular degeneration (AMD). The usefulness of omega-3 fatty acids goes beyond vision, having a wide impact on cardiovascular health.

A recent investigation proved their relevance in maintaining a healthy circulatory system and providing adequate blood flow to the fragile blood vessels of the retina.

These nutritional jewels serve as not only beautiful accompaniments to the meal but also significant sources of DHA and EPA, boosting retinal resilience with each delightful mouthful.

A recent study offers insight on the delicate balance between omega-3 and omega-6 fatty acids. While omega-3s have anti-inflammatory qualities, the excess of omega-6s in current diets may tilt the balance toward inflammation.

Finding the appropriate balance becomes vital for good retinal health and general well-being. Supplements are becoming increasingly popular among individuals who desire to enhance their omega-3 consumption. Fish oil capsules, krill oil, and algae-based supplements are all feasible choices, each with its own unique DHA and EPA profile. However, consulting a healthcare expert before increasing is crucial to guarantee tailored instruction.

Chapter 2: Breakfasts to Brighten Your Day

Sunrise Smoothie Bowl

Ingredients:

1. **Fresh fruit:** The Sunrise Smoothie Bowl's core is a combination of fresh fruits that paint the canvas of your morning. Consider mixing delicious strawberries, vibrant mango pieces, and antioxidant-rich blueberries. These fruits not only deliver a rush of natural sweetness but also feature a spectrum of vitamins, minerals, and phytonutrients that are necessary for eye health and general well-being.

2. **Leafy Greens:** A handful of leafy greens, such as spinach or kale, may increase your nutritional profile. These greens add vision-boosting lutein and zeaxanthin to your smoothie, giving it an earthy depth and enhancing its antioxidant content.

3. **Greek yogurt:** A hefty tablespoon of Greek yogurt brings out the richness. Aside from its lovely smoothness, Greek yogurt offers protein, probiotics for gut health, and a pleasant thickness that converts your smoothie into a spoon-friendly bowl.

4. **Omega-3 Boost:** Add a spoonful of chia seeds or flaxseed to the mixture. These little powerhouses give a punch of omega-3 fatty acids, improving retinal health and providing a delightful crunch to your Sunrise Smoothie Bowl.

5. **Liquid base:** Choose a liquid foundation that matches your tastes, such as almond milk, coconut water, or a dab of orange juice. These treatments not only enhance the tropical smell, but they also offer extra vitamins and minerals.

6. **Toppings:** The toppings are what give your Sunrise Smoothie Bowl its ultimate perfection. Consider adding granola for crunch, nuts for texture, and a drizzle of honey or maple syrup for sweetness.

Nutritional benefits:

1. **Vitamins and antioxidants:** The mix of fresh fruits and lush greens supplies your bowl with a range of vitamins, including Vitamin C, Vitamin A, and other antioxidants. These substances work synergistically to limit oxidative stress, boost immunological function, and promote beautiful skin and vivid eyes.

2. **Protein Power:** Greek yogurt not only adds creaminess but also delivers a big protein boost. Protein is needed for muscle repair, satiety, and sustained energy throughout the day, so your Sunrise Smoothie Bowl is a healthy breakfast option.

3. **Omega-3 Fatty Acids:** Chia seeds and flaxseeds contribute omega-3 fatty acids to your morning routine. These nutritious fats promote brain function, cardiovascular health, and, most significantly, eye and retinal health.

4. **Fiber-Rich Benefits:** The mix of fruits, vegetables, and seeds offers a high fiber content. Fiber promotes digestion, enhances satiety, and helps to maintain a healthy gut microbiota, all of which contribute to overall well-being.

In a high-speed blender, add fresh fruits, leafy greens, Greek yogurt, seeds, and your choice of liquid base.

Blend until smooth and creamy, adjusting the consistency to your preference.

Transfer the smoothie to a bowl and show your creativity by decorating with a range of scrumptious toppings. Arrange sliced strawberries, mango cubes, chia seeds, and granola in a beautifully pleasing presentation. Drizzle honey or maple syrup over your creation to give it a touch of sweetness.

Serve your sunnrise smoothie bowl straight away, allowing each mouthful to be a sensory adventure of tastes, textures, and nutritious richness.

Nutrient-Packed Overnight Oats

Ingredients:

Rolled Oats: Overnight Oats is founded on rolled oats, which are basic yet effective. These whole grains are high in fiber, which offers a continuous source of energy, helps digestive health, and adds to a sensation of fullness.

Liquid Base: Choose a liquid base that matches your activities and nutritional objectives. Almond milk, oat milk, and Greek yogurt are all rich in creaminess and contain vitamins, minerals, and microorganisms that are helpful to digestive health.

Fresh fruit: Increase your vitamin intake with a variety of fresh fruits. Berries, sliced bananas, and chopped apples are abundant in vitamins, antioxidants, and fiber, in addition to being inherently tasty.

Seeds and Nuts: Sprinkle chia seeds, flaxseeds, or sliced almonds to create a textural symphony. These components not only give a wonderful crunch, but they also deliver omega-3 fatty acids, protein, and important minerals.

Sweeteners and taste enhancers: Use natural sweeteners such as honey, maple syrup, or a dab of vanilla essence. These compounds improve sweetness without decreasing nutritive content, resulting in a well-balanced taste profile.

Nutritional Benefits:

1. **Fiber for Sustainable Energy:** The combination of rolled oats and fruits in overnight oats gives a large quantity of nutritious fiber. This vitamin encourages regular energy release, improves digestion, and promotes a sensation of fullness, making it a good option for people seeking extended vigor.

2. **Antioxidants present in fresh fruits:** The brilliant colors of fresh fruits suggest the presence of antioxidants, molecules that battle oxidative stress and enhance general health. Berries, in particular, feature a high antioxidant content, which increases the nutritional value of your meal.

3. **Omega-3 Fatty Acids with Protein:** Seeds and nuts not only add taste to a recipe, but they also supply critical nutrients. Chia seeds and flaxseeds offer omega-3 fatty acids, which are needed for heart and brain function, while almonds have protein, which stimulates muscle repair and satiety.

4. **Probiotics present in Greek yogurt:** If you utilize Greek yogurt as your liquid basis, you'll be adding probiotics. These good bacteria improve gut health, assist digestion, and contribute to the overall balance of your microbiome.

Nutritious Morning Ritual:

1. **The Basic Blend:** In a jar or container, add rolled oats and your selected liquid base. Adjust the ratio depending on your preferred consistency, whether thicker or more liquid.

2. **Fruit Ensemble:** Layer the oats with assorted fresh fruits. Experiment with additional combinations such as mixed berries, sliced bananas, and chopped apples. This not only adds natural sweetness to your oatmeal, but it also includes vitamins and antioxidants.

3. **Seed and Nut:** Sprinkle chia seeds, flaxseeds, or a handful of chopped almonds over the fruit layer. These ingredients add texture, taste, and a nutritional boost of omega-3, protein, and important minerals.

4. **The Sweetness and Flavor Finale:** Drizzle with honey, maple syrup, or add a dab of vanilla essence for additional sweetness and flavor. Stir carefully to ensure a uniform dispersion of the components.

5. **Refrigerate overnight:** Let the ensemble marinate in the refrigerator overnight. The oats absorb the liquid, the fruits blend, and the tastes build, culminating in a magnificent symphony by morning.

Superfood Omelette Delight

Ingredients:

1. **Eggs:** At the core of the Superfood Omelette is a simple but effective egg. Eggs, which are high in protein, vital amino acids, and vitamins, serve as the basis for the superfood symphony.

2. **Leafy Greens:** Enhance your omelette with nutrient-dense leafy greens like spinach, kale, or Swiss chard. These greens feature a plethora of vitamins, minerals, and antioxidants, which aid eye health and general well-being.

3. **Avocados:** Avocado slices add creaminess and a healthy fat boost. Avocados are abundant in monounsaturated fats, which enhance heart health and add a delightful texture to your omelette.

4. **Tomato:** Tomatoes not only give color but also carry lycopene, an antioxidant renowned for its ability to lessen the occurrence of chronic illnesses. Their

juiciness complements the omelette, bringing taste and nutritional benefits.

5. **Quinoa:** Cooked quinoa may offer protein and a nutty texture to your omelette. Quinoa is a complete protein source, delivering all necessary amino acids and contributing to a sensation of fullness.

6. **Feta/Goat Cheese:** A sprinkling of feta or goat cheese will improve the taste profile. These cheeses not only have a great flavor but also include calcium and other critical minerals that improve bone health.

7. **Turmeric:** Use turmeric not only for its warm, earthy taste but also for its anti-inflammatory effects. Curcumin, the major component in turmeric, adds color and possible health benefits to your Superfood Omelette.

Nutritional Benefits:

1. **Protein Power:** Eggs deliver a complete protein supply, which is required for muscle repair, satiety, and general energy. The combination of eggs, quinoa, and cheese offers a robust protein profile.

2. **Antioxidant Booster:** Leafy greens, tomatoes, and avocados contain a high concentration of antioxidants, which protect cells from oxidative stress and may lower

the incidence of chronic illnesses. The vibrant rainbow also represents a varied spectrum of vitamins and minerals.

3. **Healthy fats:** Avocado and cheese add healthy fats to the mix, improving heart health and satisfaction. These lipids, together with the protein from eggs, result in a well-balanced and fulfilling lunch.

4. **Nutrient density:** Quinoa provides not simply protein but other vital nutrients like fiber, iron, magnesium, and manganese. This superfood grain boosts the nutritional content of your omelette, supporting digestion and general well-being.

5. **Anti-inflammatory Properties:** Turmeric, with its primary component, curcumin, has anti-inflammatory benefits. This not only improves the taste, but it may also have health advantages by enhancing the body's natural defensive systems.

Creating Your Superfood Omelette:

1. **Whisk and season:** In a bowl, mix together the eggs and season with salt, pepper, and a touch of turmeric. Turmeric not only delivers a warm color but also has anti-inflammatory qualities.

2. **Sauté greens:** Cook your choice of greens in a skillet until wilted. Add tomatoes and cooked quinoa to the mixture to create a colorful and nutrient-dense basis for your omelet.

3. **Pour and Cook:** Pour the whisked eggs over the sautéed greens and allow them to set. As the edges firm up, top with slices of avocado and crumbled feta or goat cheese.

4. **Fold and serve:** When the eggs are thoroughly cooked, fold the omelette in half and allow the cheese to melt slightly. Transfer the superfood omelette to a serving platter and top with additional herbs or olive oil.

Chapter 3: Lunches for Luminous Eyes

Grilled Salmon Salad with Avocado

Ingredients:

1. **Grilled salmon:** At the center of this salad is an excellent ingredient—grilled salmon. Salmon is powerful in omega-3 fatty acids, high-quality protein, and a spectrum of critical vitamins and minerals, making it not only tasty but also good for heart health and general well-being.

2. **Avocado:** The creamy smoothness of the avocado gives a lovely touch to the salad. Avocado, which is abundant in monounsaturated fats, fiber, and vitamins, not only provides taste to meals but also improves cardiovascular health and satiety.

3. **Leafy greens:** Select a variety of leafy greens, such as spinach, arugula, or mixed baby greens. These greens have a nutrient-dense base, containing vitamins,

minerals, and antioxidants that are vital for immune support and general health.

4. **Cherry tomatoes:** Cherry tomatoes' burst of sweetness and color not only give visual appeal but also contain antioxidants such as lycopene. This chemical is widely recognized for its ability to counteract oxidative stress and increase skin health.

5. **Cucumbers:** Crisp cucumber slices make a delightful accent to the salad. Cucumbers, which are low in calories and rich in hydration, help with overall hydration while also supplying vitamins and minerals for a balanced nutritional profile.

6. **Red Onions:** Thinly sliced red onions give crispness while also supplying flavonoids and antioxidants. These chemicals are renowned for their potential to promote heart health and decrease inflammation.

7. **Lemon vinaigrette:** A mild and tangy lemon vinaigrette is the right dressing. Lemon not only tastes great, but it also includes vitamin C, which is believed to enhance the immune system.

Nutritional Benefits:

1. **Omega-3 Fatty Acids Promote Heart Health:** Grilled salmon, which is high in omega-3 fatty acids, supports cardiovascular health by maintaining good cholesterol levels, decreasing inflammation, and maybe lowering the risk of heart disease.

2. **Monounsaturated Fats Promote Satiety:** Avocado's monounsaturated fats give a rich and creamy texture, giving a sensation of fullness. These good fats enhance satiety and may assist in weight control.

3. **Nutrient Density of Leafy Greens:** Leafy greens are filled with nutrients like vitamins A, C, and K, as well as folate and iron. Their low calorie count, combined with their excellent nutritional value, makes them an important element of a well-balanced diet.

4. **Antioxidants Promote Cellular Health:** Cherry tomatoes, cucumbers, and red onions deliver a range of antioxidants. These substances battle oxidative stress, promote cellular health, and may lessen the risk of chronic illnesses.

5. **Lean Protein Promotes Muscle Health:** Grilled salmon contains high-quality protein, which is needed for muscle repair, maintenance, and general cellular

function. Including lean protein in the salad creates a well-balanced and delicious lunch.

Creating Your Grilled Salmon Salad:

1. **Grilling salmon:** Season the salmon with your choice of herbs and spices. Grill until the fish is flaky with a slightly browned surface.

2. **Making the Salad:** In a large bowl, add the leafy greens, cherry tomatoes, cucumber slices, and thinly sliced red onions. Gently blend the ingredients to make a rich and bright foundation.

3. **Add the cooked salmon:** Place the grilled salmon on top of the greens. Break it into flaky bits or leave it as a fillet, depending on your desire.

4. **Slicing avocados:** Slice the avocado and spread the creamy parts over the salad. The avocado not only provides richness, but it also improves the taste of the grilled salmon.

5. **Drizzled Lemon Vinaigrette:** Create a simple lemon vinaigrette by blending fresh lemon juice, olive oil, salt,

and pepper. Drizzle the vinaigrette over the salad to produce a light and refreshing covering.

6. **Garnish and serve:** Garnish the salad with extra herbs, such as dill or parsley, for a burst of flavor. Serve immediately to let the flavors mingle and create a symphony of taste and texture.

Quinoa and Vegetable Power Bowl

Ingredients:

1. **Quinoa:** This power bowl is based on quinoa, a gluten-free whole grain packed with protein, fiber, and important vitamins and minerals. Its adaptability makes it the perfect basis for a nutrient-dense meal.

2. **Colorful Vegetables:** A rainbow of vibrant veggies, including bell peppers, cherry tomatoes, broccoli, and carrots, create the basis of this power bowl. Each vegetable adds its own unique blend of vitamins, antioxidants, and fiber.

3. **Leafy greens:** Incorporate nutrient-dense leafy greens such as spinach, kale, and Swiss chard.

These greens contain a spectrum of vitamins, minerals, and phytonutrients, improving the nutritional value of the power bowl.

4. **Avocados:** Creamy avocado slices not only increase texture, but they also provide heart-healthy monounsaturated fats, vitamins, and minerals. Avocado lends a bit of refinement to the power bowl. 5

5. **Chickpeas/Edamame:** Chickpeas or edamame may be added to boost the protein content. These plant-based proteins supply vital amino acids for muscle health and sustained energy.

6. **Nuts or Seeds:** Fill the power bowl with a variety of nuts or seeds, such as almonds, pumpkin seeds, and sunflower seeds. These supplements deliver crunch, healthy fats, and a dose of important minerals.

7. **Dress:** A light and pleasant dressing prepared with olive oil, lemon juice, and a splash of herbs may bind the components together, increasing the overall taste while delivering extra vital fats.

Nutritional Benefits:

1. **Complete Protein Source:** Quinoa stands itself as a complete protein source, comprising all nine necessary amino acids. This makes the Quinoa and Vegetable Power Bowl an ideal alternative for those seeking plant-based protein sources.

2. **Fiber-Rich Benefits:** The combination of quinoa, veggies, and legumes delivers a considerable quantity of beneficial fiber. Fiber enhances digestive health, assists in weight control, and adds to a sensation of fullness.

3. **Antioxidant-rich Vegetables:** The diversity of bright veggies adds a depth of antioxidants to the power bowl. Antioxidants minimize oxidative stress, possibly lowering the risk of chronic illnesses and enhancing general health.

4. **Healthy Fats from Avocados:** Avocados include heart-healthy monounsaturated fats that not only improve the creaminess of the dish but also give satiety and support cardiovascular health.

5. **Plant-Based Protein:** Chickpeas and edamame are plant-based protein sources,

making them an ideal alternative for individuals searching for a variety. These proteins enhance muscle health and provide sustained energy.

6. **Essential Nutrients in Nuts and Seeds:** Nuts or seeds added to the power bowl supply critical elements like magnesium, zinc, and iron. They also contain healthy fats, resulting in a delightful crunch and nutritional benefits.

Creating Your Quinoa and Vegetable Power Bowl:

1. **How to Cook Quinoa:** Rinse the quinoa carefully and cook according to package directions. After cooking, fluff it with a fork to achieve a light and fluffy texture.

2. **Roasting vegetables:** Toss veggies in olive oil, then season with herbs and spices of your preference. Roast until golden brown. Roasting boosts the taste and texture of veggies.

3. **Assembly of the Bowl:** In a big bowl, prepare a liberal quantity of cooked quinoa. Arrange the roasted veggies, avocado slices, chickpeas or edamame, and a sprinkle of nuts or seeds.

4. **Drizzle the Dressing:** Create a simple dressing by blending olive oil, lemon juice, salt, and pepper. Drizzle the dressing over the power bowl, maintaining a uniform coating.

5. **Garnish:** Garnish the power bowl with fresh herbs, such as parsley or cilantro, for a blast of flavor and depth.

6. **Serve and enjoy:** Serve the quinoa and vegetable power bowl straight away, allowing the flavors to combine and create a gourmet experience that delights the senses while nourishing the body.

Spinach and Blueberry Salad with Walnut Vinaigrette

Ingredients:

1. **Fresh spinach:** Fresh spinach, which is nutrient-dense and vitamin-rich, acts as the salad's base. Spinach offers a sturdy basis, rich with iron, calcium, and a plethora of vitamins A and K.

2. **Sweet blueberries:** Blueberries' burst of sweetness and brilliant color not only make a stunning contrast, but they also contain antioxidants, notably anthocyanins, which are renowned for their potential health benefits.

3. **Crunchy walnuts:** Walnuts, with their earthy taste and delicious crunch, offer heart-healthy monounsaturated fats and omega-3 fatty acids to the meal. These nuts boost not only the flavor but also the overall well-being. 4. **Feta/Goat Cheese:** Add extra feta or goat cheese for a savory taste and creamy texture. These cheeses add calcium, protein, and a burst of flavor to counter the sweetness of the blueberries.

5. **Red Onions:** Thinly sliced red onion provides pungency and color. Red onion contains antioxidants and chemicals that may have health advantages, in addition to its culinary appeal.

6. **Avocado slices:** Avocado slices offer a creamy smoothness to the salad while also supplying essential monounsaturated fats, vitamins, and minerals.

Nutritional Benefits:

1. **Antioxidant Boost from Blueberries:** Blueberries, which are abundant in antioxidants, play a vital role in

countering oxidative stress. Blueberries have anthocyanins, which benefit heart health, cognitive function, and general well-being.

2. **Iron and Vitamin K in Spinach:** Fresh spinach contains a high content of iron, which is needed for oxygen transport in the body. Additionally, the high vitamin K concentration helps bone health and blood coagulation.

3. **Omega-3 Fatty Acids for Heart Health:** Walnuts provide omega-3 fatty acids, which support heart health and may lower inflammation. Including walnuts in the salad provides a layer of nutritional richness.

4. **Protein and Calcium in Cheese:** Feta or goat cheese provides protein and calcium to the salad. Protein increases muscular performance, while calcium is needed for bone strength and general health.

5. **Avocado delivers healthful fats and creaminess:** Avocado's creamy texture enriches the salad's overall mouthfeel, giving crucial monounsaturated fats, vitamins, and minerals that promote satiety and cardiovascular health.

6. **Dietary fiber:** The mix of spinach, blueberries, and other ingredients gives a wonderful amount of healthy

fiber. Fiber supports digestive health, helps to maintain a healthy weight, and offers a sensation of fullness.

Creating Your Salad:

1. **Preparing the ingredients:** Wash and dry the fresh spinach properly. Rinse the blueberries, finely slice the red onion, crumble the cheese, and cut the avocado into slices. Roast the walnuts for an added depth of flavor.

2. **Making the Salad:** In a large bowl, mix the fresh spinach, blueberries, red onion slices, crumbled cheese, avocado slices, and toasted walnuts. Lightly toss the ingredients to make a visually beautiful and balanced ensemble.

3. **Drizzle the walnut vinaigrette:** Create a simple walnut vinaigrette by blending walnut oil, balsamic vinegar, Dijon mustard, honey, salt, and pepper. Drizzle the vinaigrette over the salad, ensuring that each component is gently covered.

4. **Toss and garnish:** Gently toss the salad to properly spread the vinaigrette. For an added blast of flavor, sprinkle with more roasted walnuts and fresh herbs like mint or basil.

5. **Serve and enjoy:** Serve the spinach and blueberry salad with walnut vinaigrette immediately to let the flavors blend. Enjoy this stimulating symphony of tastes, textures, and nutritional benefits as a single meal or as a lovely side dish.

Chapter 4: Dinner Dishes for Clear Vision

Baked Cod with Lemon and Herbs

Ingredients:

1. **Cod Fillets:** At the core of this recipe are clean cod fillets, a lean and mild fish that acts as a flexible canvas for absorbing the complimentary tastes of lemon and herbs. Select high-quality, fresh fish for the greatest flavor and texture.

2. **Fresh lemons:** The strong citrus smells of fresh lemons lend a zesty freshness to the fish. The acidity not only increases the taste profile, but it also offers a refreshing aspect that balances the fish's richness.

3. **Aromatic herbs (such as parsley, dill, and thyme):** An assortment of fresh herbs adds a delightful flavor to the fish. Parsley, dill, and thyme, for example, produce a symphony of tastes, ranging from earthy and slightly sweet to

bright and lemony, improving the overall gourmet experience.

4. **Garlic cloves:** Garlic, with its wonderful and sometimes pungent overtones, gives richness to the cuisine. Garlic, whether minced or sliced, enhances the mildness of fish and adds to its overall richness.

5. **Olive oils:** The marinade's base is built of high-quality olive oil, which offers a delectable covering for the cod. It not only gives the fish a rich taste, but it also keeps it wet during baking.

6. **Salt and pepper:** Salt and pepper are the cornerstones of seasoning. They bring out the inherent tastes of the fish while enhancing the herbal and citrus undertones.

Cooking Techniques:

1. **Marinate the cod:** Begin by marinating the cod fillets in olive oil, fresh lemon juice, minced garlic, chopped herbs, salt, and pepper. Allow the cod to marinade for at least 30 minutes so that the spices may penetrate the fish.

2. **Preheat the oven:** Preheat the oven to the right temperature, generally approximately 375°F (190°C). Ensure that the oven is appropriately preheated for uniform cooking and a golden finish.

3. **Baking Cod:** Place the marinated fish fillets on a baking pan lined with parchment paper. Bake the fish in the preheated oven until it is opaque and easily flaked with a fork. The baking time may vary depending on the thickness of the fillets.

4. **Broiling to a Golden Finish:** Broil the fish for the final few minutes to produce a golden finish and a little crispiness on the edges. This strategy boosts the meal's visual beauty while also offering tactile depth.

5. **Garnish with fresh herbs:** Finish by topping the grilled fish with extra fresh herbs. This not only gives a flash of color but also accentuates the herbal infusion, giving it a visually pleasing appearance.

6. **Serve with lemon wedges:** Serve baked cod with lemon and herbs, with fresh lemon slices on

the side. A squeeze of lemon soon before tasting the cuisine improves the zesty undertones and brightens the overall taste.

Nutritional Advantages:

1. **Lean Protein from Cod:** Cod is a low-fat, high-quality protein source that is needed for muscle repair, maintenance, and general cell function. It provides a tasty and healthy base for a balanced meal.

2. **Omega-3 Fatty Acids:** Cod is noted for its high level of omega-3 fatty acids, which support heart health, cognitive function, and inflammation reduction. Cod in the diet supports overall cardiovascular health.

3. **Antioxidants obtained from herbs and lemon:** Fresh herbs and lemon give antioxidants to the meal. These chemicals minimize oxidative stress, potentially lowering the risk of chronic illnesses and increasing general health.

4. **Low-calorie and nutrient-dense:** Baked fish with lemon and herbs is a low-calorie alternative that does not sacrifice nutritional value. It

contains critical vitamins and minerals without adding calories, making it a perfect option for health-conscious clients.

Roasted Vegetable and Chickpea Stew

Ingredients:

1. **Mixed veggies (such as carrots, bell peppers, zucchini, and sweet potatoes):** A broad mix of veggies serves as the base of this stew. Each has its own particular taste, texture, and vitamin and mineral profile.

2. **Chickpeas, canned or cooked:** Chickpeas are a protein powerhouse, giving a substantial and fulfilling ingredient to the stew. They also have a nutty taste and nutritional fiber to aid digestive health.

3. **Onion with Garlic:** The fragrant duet of onions and garlic serves as the stew's delectable basis. They add depth and richness, increasing the overall taste profile.

4. **Vegetable broth:** The stew's base is produced with high-quality vegetable broth, which infuses a rich liquid

that blends the flavors together. Choose a low-sodium option for extra control over the dish's salt level.

5. **Herbs and spices (such as thyme, rosemary, and paprika):** A combination of herbs and spices lends warmth and depth to the stew. Thyme and rosemary create an earthy taste, while paprika provides smokiness and depth.

6. **Olive oils:** Olive oil serves two purposes: it coats the veggies for roasting and gives the stew a rich texture. Its monounsaturated fats also have heart-healthy characteristics.

7. **Tomatoes, canned or fresh:** Tomatoes lend acidity and a sense of umami to the stew. Using canned or fresh tomatoes boosts the overall richness of flavor.

Techniques:

1. **Roasting vegetables:** Begin by frying the different veggies in olive oil until they are golden brown. This stage intensifies the flavors and adds depth to the entire stew.

2. **Sauté Onions and Garlic:** In a large saucepan, sauté finely chopped onions and minced garlic until

translucent. This makes for an excellent basis for the stew.

3. **Combining Roasted Vegetables with Chickpeas:** Add the roasted veggies and chickpeas to the saucepan and stir with the sautéed onions and garlic. This approach ensures that each component absorbs the tastes of the others.

4. **Pour Vegetable Broth:** Pour in the vegetable broth to make a lovely liquid that binds the stew together. Adjust the amount of stock to your desired stew consistency.

5. **Seasoning with herbs and spices:** Incorporate a variety of herbs and spices, such as thyme, rosemary, and paprika, into the stew. Season to taste with salt and pepper, then leave the flavors to blend and develop over medium heat.

6. **Add Tomatoes:** Depending on your tastes and seasonal availability, use canned or fresh tomatoes. Tomatoes lend acidity and depth to the stew, which boosts its overall complexity.

7. **Simmering to perfection:** Allow the stew to simmer over low heat for the flavors to blend and deepen. This simmering time also guarantees that the veggies and chickpeas absorb the delicious richness of the broth.

Nutritional Benefits:

1. **Plant-Based Protein from Chickpeas:** Chickpeas offer a plant-based protein supply, promoting muscular health and producing a flavorful and nutrient-dense stew.

2. **Dietary Fiber and Digestive Health:** Chickpeas, when paired with the diversity of vegetables, offer vital fiber. This enhances digestive health, helps to maintain a healthy weight, and provides you with a sensation of fullness.

3. **Vitamins and minerals found in vegetables:** The broad range of roasted veggies provides a variety of vitamins and minerals, including vitamin A, vitamin C, potassium, and folate, which support general well-being.

4. **Monounsaturated lipids are heart-healthy:** Olive oil, a major ingredient, contributes heart-healthy monounsaturated fats to the stew. These fats help cardiovascular health and boost the overall richness of the meal.

5. **Antioxidants present in herbs and tomatoes:** The stew's herbs and tomatoes provide a range of antioxidants, which serve to counteract oxidative stress and may minimize the onset of chronic illnesses.

Stir-Fried Tofu and Broccoli with Sesame

Ingredients:

1. **Firm tofu:** The major component in this stir-fry is firm tofu, a flexible plant-based protein source. Tofu absorbs the rich fragrances from the stir-fry while maintaining a delicate and pleasing texture.

2. **Fresh broccoli florets:** Broccoli, with its brilliant green hue, provides a cruciferous crunch to the meal. Broccoli is rich in vitamins, minerals, and fiber, which adds to its total nutritional worth.

3. **Sesame oil:** lends a unique nutty taste to the stir-fry, improving the overall depth of flavor. It also contains heart-healthy monounsaturated fats and a lovely scent.

4. **Soy Sauce (or Tamari for a gluten-free alternative):** Soy sauce gives the delicious umami undertones required for stir-fry. Tamari may be used as a gluten-free substitute without affecting taste.

5. **Garlic and Ginger**: A blend of garlic and ginger lends fragrant richness to the meal. Their savory and spicy scents add complexity to the stir-fry.

6. **Sesame Seed:** Toasted sesame seeds offer a lovely crunch and nuttiness to the stir-fry. They also bring extra levels of taste and visual appeal.

7. **Green onions:** Fresh green onions give a light onion taste and a burst of color. They act as a garnish, providing a touch of freshness to the completed meal.

Techniques:

1. **Pressing and cubing tofu:** Begin by pressing the firm tofu to eliminate extra moisture. After pressing, cut the tofu into bite-sized pieces. This approach results in a harder texture and greater flavor absorption during stir-frying.

2. **Blanching broccoli:** To keep the broccoli florets vividly colored and fresh, blanch them quickly in boiling water. This step also begins the cooking process, so the broccoli cooks evenly throughout the stir-frying.

3. **Preparing Aromatics:** Sauté the chopped garlic and ginger in sesame oil over medium heat until fragrant.

This makes a fragrant basis for the stir-fry, infusing it with savory and spicy tastes.

4. **Adding Tofu and Broccoli:** Add the cubed tofu and the blanched broccoli to the pan. Stir-fry them together until the tofu acquires a golden crust and the broccoli absorbs the delightful fragrances.

5. **Drizzle with soy sauce:** Drizzle soy sauce evenly over the tofu and broccoli. The soy sauce provides culinary depth to the meal and caramelizes the items wonderfully. 6. **Sprinkle Sesame Seeds:** Sprinkle toasted sesame seeds over the stir-fry. The seeds create a nice crunch and enhance the nutty taste character.

7. Garnish with green onions. Finish the stir-fry by garnishing with finely chopped green onions. This process gives a touch of freshness and visual appeal to the entire meal.

Nutritional Advantages:

1. **Plant-Based Protein from Tofu:** Tofu is a great plant-based protein source that includes vital amino acids for muscle function and general health.

2. **Fiber and Vitamins in Broccoli:** Broccoli offers dietary fiber, vitamins C and K, and a range of

antioxidants. These nutrients aid digestion, immunological function, and general health.

3. **Healthful Fats from Sesame Oil:** Sesame oil includes heart-healthy monounsaturated fats, which increase the richness of the meal and help cardiovascular health.

4. **Umami Flavor of Soy Sauce:** Soy sauce offers the umami taste vital for stir-fries. It adds depth and flavor to the meal while maintaining its plant-based foundation.

5. **Nutritious Sesame Seeds:** Toasted sesame seeds provide vital minerals like copper, manganese, and iron. They also contain healthy fats, which provide nutrition and texture to the stir-fry.

Chapter 5: Snacks for Sharp Sight

Crunchy Carrot Sticks with Hummus

Ingredients:

1. **Fresh carrot sticks:** Fresh carrot sticks are the highlight of this snack, with their gorgeous orange hue. Carrots have a natural sweetness and delicious texture, making them great for dipping into hummus.

2. **Hummus (storebought or homemade):** Hummus, a creamy dip prepared with chickpeas, tahini, olive oil, lemon juice, and garlic, works beautifully with the carrots. Hummus, whether store-bought or homemade, offers a range of tastes and plant-based nutrients for the snacking experience.

3. **Extra Virgin Olive Oil:** A sprinkle of extra virgin olive oil over the hummus enriches its velvety texture while also supplying heart-healthy monounsaturated fats, imparting a subtle richness to each mouthful.

4. **Fresh lemon juice:** The zesty tones of fresh lemon juice add a blast of lemony sharpness to the hummus, cutting through the creaminess and complimenting the sweetness of the carrots.

5. **Garlic cloves:** Minced garlic cloves offer a savory flavor to the hummus, which contrasts beautifully with the carrots' innate sweetness.

6. **Paprika or Smoked Paprika (optional):** For those who appreciate the taste of smokiness, adding paprika or smoked paprika to the hummus gives it a delicate and subtle flavor layer. Sensory

Texture and Flavors:

1. **Crunchy carrot sticks:** Fresh carrot sticks have a beautiful crunch, providing a sensory symphony that pleases the palate. The process of dipping and biting into the sharpness of the carrots results in a dynamic and delightful texture.

2) **Creamy Hummus:** Hummus, with its velvety smoothness, gives a delightful and creamy feel to the snack. Its taste profile, a beautiful combination of chickpeas, tahini, and garlic, enhances the carrots' inherent sweetness.

3. **Zesty Lemon with Savory Garlic:** Fresh lemon juice and minced garlic offer a zesty freshness to the hummus while also providing great depth. These additives improve the overall taste experience, making each dip a joy.

4. **Olive Oil Elegance:** A trickle of extra virgin olive oil not only enriches the texture of the hummus but also offers a subtle richness that links the entire snack together.

5. **Optional paprika infusion:** For those searching for taste diversity, paprika or smoked paprika adds a little smokiness to the hummus, giving it additional richness and depth.

Nutritional Benefits:

1. **Carrots provide beta-carotene and fiber:** Carrots, abundant in beta-carotene, support eye health and contain dietary fiber, which assists digestion. The crunchiness supports jaw health and enjoyment.

2. **Hummus includes plant-based protein and fiber:** Hummus prepared from chickpeas delivers plant-based protein and fiber. This combination encourages fullness,

making the snack a good option for people seeking both nourishment and amusement.

3. **Olive oil provides heart-healthy lipids:** The drizzle of extra virgin olive oil over the hummus includes heart-healthy monounsaturated fats. These fats boost cardiovascular health and add a touch of refinement to the snack.

4. **Antioxidants and Vitamin C:** Fresh lemon juice not only increases taste, but it also includes antioxidants and vitamin C. These components help with immune support and general well-being.

5. **Optional paprika for taste and antioxidants:** The use of paprika or smoked paprika not only improves taste but also delivers antioxidants. This optional feature adds a degree of complexity and possible health advantages.

Trail Mix with Nuts and Dried Berries

Ingredients:

1. **Almonds:** This trail mix is based on almonds, a crispy and nutrient-dense nut that delivers a

terrific protein and healthy fat boost. Almonds have a robust bulk and a delicate flavor.

2. **Walnuts:** add a characteristic earthy taste as well as omega-3 fatty acids to the trail mix, boosting its nutritional value. Their deep, almost bitter fragrances add depth to each taste.

3. **Cashews:** Cashews give a creamy texture and subtle sweetness, which contrast nicely with the crunchier nuts in the mix. They provide healthy fats, protein, and important minerals.

4. **Pistachio:** give a splash of brilliant green and a distinct taste to the mix. These nuts are not only great, but they also provide added fiber and minerals.

5. **Dried Cranberries:** The acidity of dried cranberries lends flavor and chewiness to the mix. Cranberries also provide antioxidants and a hint of natural sweetness.

6. **Dried blueberries:** Blueberries in their dried form give a sweet and tart layer to the trail mix. Dried blueberries are abundant in antioxidants, which enhance general health.

7. **Golden raisins:** Golden raisins have a natural sweetness and chewy texture. They complement the other dried berries, bringing a touch of warmth to the combination.

8. **Dark chocolate chips (optional):** For persons with a sweet appetite, dark chocolate chips may be employed in moderation. Dark chocolate delivers antioxidants and a sensation of pleasure without overpowering the combination with sugar.

Nutritional Benefits:

1. **Nuts provide protein and healthy fats:** Almonds, walnuts, cashews, and pistachios offer a balanced combination of protein, monounsaturated fats, and omega-3 fatty acids. This trio enhances satiety, cardiovascular health, and general well-being.

2. **Antioxidants present in Berries:** Dried cranberries and blueberries are abundant in antioxidants, which help battle oxidative stress and may lower the risk of chronic illnesses.

These berries add a flare of color and taste to the combination.

3. **Fiber Promotes Satiety:** Nuts and dried berries provide nutritional fiber, boost digestive health, and give a tasty flavor to the trail mix. Fiber creates a sensation of fullness, making the combination a great snack for busy lives.

4. **Essential Minerals:** Cashews and pistachios supply vital nutrients like magnesium, phosphorus, and potassium. These minerals serve critical roles in bone health, energy metabolism, and general cell function.

5. **Natural sugars from dried fruit:** dried cranberries, blueberries, and golden raisins all contain natural sugars, giving a sweet component without the need for extra refined sweeteners. This natural sweetness enriches the entire taste profile.

6. **Dark Chocolate Antioxidant (Optional):** Dark chocolate chips have flavonoids, which are antioxidants. Dark chocolate in moderation may have cardiovascular advantages and offer a lovely touch of enjoyment.

Customization and Serving Suggestions:

1. **Mix and match:** The variety of Trail Mix with Nuts and Dried Berries is what makes it so enticing. Feel free to modify the ratio of nuts to dried berries to suit your tastes. Experiment with various nuts and dried fruits to discover a mix that matches your taste.

2. **Portion control:** Although trail mix is a nutrient-dense snack, it is vital to exercise portion management. To minimize overindulging and make on-the-go eating simpler, divide the mixture into snack-sized bags or containers ahead of time.

3. **On the Go Snacking:** Carry a tiny quantity of trail mix in a resealable bag for a fast and energy-boosting snack for outdoor activities, work, or travel. The mix's mobility makes it a simple and gratifying option in a range of circumstances.

Greek Yogurt Parfait with Berries

Ingredients:

1. **Greek yogurt (full or reduced fat):** This parfait's basis is Greek yogurt, which is heavy in protein and creamy. Depending on your tastes, you may pick between full-fat and low-fat varieties, both of which have a thick texture. 2. **Fresh Berries (such as strawberries, blueberries, and raspberries):** A trio of fresh berries provides color, sweetness, and antioxidants. Strawberries bring juiciness, blueberries provide a touch of acidity, and raspberries provide a brilliant color and unusual texture. 3. **Honey or maple syrup:** A dusting of honey or maple syrup provides a bit of natural sweetness to the parfait. This procedure increases the overall taste profile while maintaining the natural deliciousness of the components. 4. **Granola (optional):** Add your favorite granola for a great crunch and texture. Choose a flavor that complements the richness of the Greek yogurt and provides a pleasant aspect to each taste.

5. **Chia seed (optional):** Chia seeds give a nutritional boost by delivering omega-3 fatty acids and adding texture. When soaked, chia seeds develop a gel-like consistency that lends a delightful chewiness to the parfait.

6. **Vanilla extract (optional):** add a dab of pure vanilla essence to the Greek yogurt to add more taste. This small ingredient increases the parfait's overall richness and scent.

Techniques:

1. **The bottom layer of Greek yogurt:** Start by spooning a layer of Greek yogurt into the bottom of a serving glass or plate. The thickness of this layer may be modified according to personal choice.

2. **Drizzle with honey or maple syrup:** Sprinkle a little honey or maple syrup over the Greek yogurt layer. This stage delivers a sensation of sweetness, which enriches the entire taste experience.

3. **Fresh Berry Layer:** Spread a thick layer of fresh berries over the Greek yogurt. Distribute the berries equally, producing a visually pleasing and colorful strata.

4. **Optional coating of chia seeds:** If using chia seeds, add 1 teaspoon over the berry layer. The seeds will absorb moisture from the yogurt and berries, resulting in a textured, nutrient-dense coating.

5. **Repeat the stacking:** Repeat the layering technique by adding another layer of Greek yogurt, then honey or

maple syrup, fresh berries, and optional granola. Continue stacking until the serving basin is full.

6. **Top with berries and granola:** Finish the parfait by topping it with a visually pleasing arrangement of fresh berries and granola. This finishing addition offers a flash of color and a delightful crunch.

Nutritional Benefits:

1. **Protein-rich Greek Yogurt:** Greek yogurt contains a high quantity of protein, which is vital for muscular function, satiety, and general health. It has a creamy texture while offering a lovely and healthy basis.

2. **Antioxidant-rich fresh berries:** The trio of fresh berries—strawberries, blueberries, and raspberries—deliver a range of antioxidants. These compounds withstand oxidative damage and support cellular health.

3. **Natural sweeteners:** honey or maple syrup give natural sweetness, removing the need for refined sweeteners. This option enriches the overall flavor by delivering extra antioxidants and trace minerals.

4. **Fiber and Nutrients in Granola:** Granola, if included, offers nutritional fiber, vitamins, and minerals.

It gives a delicious crunch and heightens the richness of the Greek yogurt.

5. **Omega-3 Fatty Acids Found in Chia Seeds:** Chia seeds, if included, give a dose of omega-3 fatty acids, which benefits heart health and adds texture to the parfait.

Chapter 6: Sweet Treats for Healthy Eyes

Dark Chocolate and Berry Bliss Bites

Ingredients:

1. **Dark chocolate (70% cocoa or more):** Dark chocolate, which is recognized for its high cocoa content, acts as the base for these joyful bits. Choose chocolate with 70% cocoa or greater, as it has a rich flavor and possible health advantages, including antioxidants.

2. **Mixed Berries (including strawberries, blueberries, and raspberries):** Fresh berries add a flash of color, natural sweetness, and antioxidants. Strawberries contribute juiciness, blueberries add a little acidity, and raspberries give a bright tint.

3. **Almonds or walnuts (optional):** Finely chopped almonds or walnuts may lend texture and a nutty depth to dishes. These nuts not only give crunch, but they also contain nutritious fats and other nutrients.

4. **Unsweetened shredded coconut (optional):** Unsweetened shredded coconut may be added to offer a tropical taste and a touch of sweetness. This optional ingredient enhances the dark chocolate and berries while offering a lovely texture.

5. **Honey or maple syrup:** A dusting of honey or maple syrup acts as a natural sweetener, improving the overall sweetness of the pleasure bits. This choice delivers a touch of enjoyment without depending on manufactured sweets.

Techniques:

1. **Melting and tempering dark chocolate:** Begin by melting the dark chocolate over a double boiler or in the microwave until smooth and glossy. Tempering the chocolate is vital for a gorgeous finish and a satisfying snap when bitten into.

2. **Dipped and Coated Berries:** Dip each fresh fruit into the melting dark chocolate, producing uniform coverage.

This process makes a wonderful chocolate shell around the fruit. Set the coated berries on a parchment-lined pan.

3. **Drizzle with honey or maple syrup:** Drizzle honey or maple syrup over the chocolate-coated berries while they are still setting. This gives an additional layer of sweetness and a glossy finish to the bites.

4. **Optional Nut and Coconut Coating:** For extra texture and taste, roll the chocolate-coated berries in finely chopped almonds or walnuts and unsweetened shredded coconut. This stage gives it a wonderful crunch with a nutty or coconut undertone.

5. **Chill to Set:** Place the completed happy pieces in the refrigerator to permit the chocolate coating to set fully. This offers a hard and pleasant sensation when biting into the exquisite delicacy.

Nutritional Benefits:

1. **Antioxidant-rich Dark Chocolate:** Dark chocolate with high cocoa content includes antioxidants, notably flavonoids, which may enhance heart health and general

well-being. It provides a wonderful and rich chocolate taste to the pleasure bites.

2. **Berries as Vitamins and Antioxidants:** Mixed berries provide a range of vitamins, minerals, and antioxidants. These chemicals increase immunological function, decrease oxidative stress, and deliver a surge of natural sweetness.

3. **Nuts provide nutritious lipids and protein:** Chopped almonds or walnuts, when combined with, give healthful fats, protein, and other nutrients. These nuts create a delightful crunch while also improving the nutritive content of the nibbles.

4. **Natural sweeteners:** Honey or maple syrup, when handled appropriately, operate as natural sweeteners, delivering sweetness without depending on synthetic sugar. This selection delivers a sensation of pleasure while retaining a balance of tastes.

5. **Fiber from Berries and Coconuts:** Berries and optional shredded coconut offer nutritional fiber, which helps digestive health and provides a sense of fullness. The fiber content gives a nutritious component to the pleasure bites.

Mango and Kiwi Sorbet

Ingredients:

1. **Ripe mangoes:** Ripe mangoes' golden richness serves as the backbone for this sorbet. Choose mangoes that are completely ripe for a powerful and natural sweetness that enriches the entire taste profile.

2. **Fresh Kiwis:** Kiwi, with its vivid green flesh and acidic taste, offers a delightful and slightly tart contrast to the sweetness of mangoes. Choose ripe but firm kiwis for the greatest texture and taste.

3. **Simple Syrup:** Sweetener is a simple syrup comprised of equal parts water and sugar. This results in a smooth and scoopable sorbet texture that lacks the grittiness of undissolved sugar.

4. **Fresh lime juice:** Fresh lime juice brightens the sorbet, giving it a zesty citrus flavor that contributes to its overall freshness. It also has a little acidity that complements the sweetness.

5. **Mint leaves (optional):** Finely chopped mint leaves may offer a sensation of herbal freshness. This optional addition complements the tropical aromas and offers a pleasant experience with each mouthful.

Techniques:

1. **Peeling and slicing mangos:** Peel and slice the ripe mangos. The purpose is to extract the flesh from the pit so that only the sweet, exquisite mango meat is utilized in the sorbet.

2. **Peeling and slicing Kiwi:** Peel and cut fresh Kiwi into rounds or slices. The slices offer visual appeal to the sorbet, and the kiwi's sharpness complements the mango's sweetness.

3. **Blend the Fruits:** In a blender, mix the chopped mangos, sliced kiwi, simple syrup, and fresh lime juice. Blend until smooth and creamy, producing a homogenous combination that preserves the tastes of both fruits.

4. **Strain (optional):** To create a smoother sorbet texture, sift the blended ingredients to eliminate any fibrous or seedy residues. This stage is optional and depends on personal taste for texture.

5. **Churning and freezing:** Transfer the mixed ingredients to an ice cream maker and churn according to the manufacturer's directions. Churning absorbs air, resulting in a light and fluffy texture. Alternatively, pour

the mixture into a small pan and freeze, stirring every 30 minutes for several hours.

6. **Garnish with mint (optional):** Once the sorbet has achieved the proper consistency, scoop it onto serving plates or cones. Garnish with finely chopped mint leaves for a flash of color and an added dose of freshness.

Nutritional benefits:

1. Vitamin C from mango and kiwi Mangoes and kiwis are abundant in vitamin C, a potent antioxidant that enhances immune health and skin vibrancy. Sorbet is a pleasant and tasty approach to enhancing vitamin C consumption.

2. **Natural sugars from fruits:** The sweetness of the sorbet derives from the natural sugars contained in mangoes and kiwis. This natural sweetness gives guilt-free enjoyment without the need for excessive additional sweets.

3. **Hydration from fruits:** Mangoes and kiwis both contain a lot of water, which helps you stay hydrated. On a hot day, eating sorbet is both a delicious and hydrating experience.

4. **Fiber Promotes Digestive Health:** The fiber in both fruits adds weight to the sorbet, boosting digestive health. Fiber helps to retain the sensation of fullness and promotes a healthy digestive system.

5. **Antioxidants for Overall Wellness:** The combination of mangoes and kiwis offers various antioxidants, including beta-carotene and quercetin. These antioxidants battle oxidative stress and promote general well-being.

Almond and Date Energy Bars

Ingredients:

1. **Almonds:** At the core of these energy bars are almonds, a nutrient-dense powerhouse. Almonds give a pleasant crunch, healthy fats, and a plethora of vitamins and minerals, including vitamin E and magnesium.

2. **Medjool Dates:** Medjool dates supply the natural sweetness and binding factor in the bars. Dates are abundant in fiber, potassium, and

natural sugars, which give sweetness while also promoting digestive health.

3. **Rolled oats:** Rolled oats offer a healthy and fiber-rich basis, giving the bars a chewy texture. Oats offer sustained energy release, making them a good element for long-term satiety.

4. **Chia seed:** Chia seeds are a nutritional powerhouse, providing omega-3 fatty acids, fiber, and texture to the bars. These little seeds boost heart health and general well-being.

5. **Almond butter:** Almond butter not only enriches the nutty taste, but it also helps the bars' cohesiveness. It boasts nutritious fats, protein, and a velvety texture that complements the crunch of almonds.

6. **Vanilla extract:** A dab of pure vanilla extract enriches the taste profile, providing warmth and sweetness. This extra addition boosts the overall flavor without overwhelming the underlying deliciousness.

7. **Sea salt:** A sprinkling of sea salt balances the sweetness and increases the depth of flavor. This

basic ingredient gives a savory tone that complements the richness of almonds and dates.

Techniques:

1. **Blending almonds and oats:** Begin by mixing almonds and rolled oats in a food processor until a coarse, crumbly texture is produced. This combination produces the bars' sturdy and nutrient-dense base.

2. **Combining Dates with Almond Butter:** Combine pitted Medjool dates and almond butter with the combined almond and oat mixture. Process until all of the ingredients are incorporated and the dough is sticky and cohesive.

3. **Add Chia Seeds and Vanilla Extract:** Add the chia seeds and, if preferred, a dab of vanilla essence to the mixture. Pulse briefly to evenly integrate these components, resulting in a well-balanced taste and texture.

4. **Pressing into the Pan:** Transfer the dough to a parchment-lined pan and push down hard to achieve a uniform layer. Use the back of a spoon

or a spatula to produce a compact and smooth surface.

5. **Chill to Set:** Place the pan in the refrigerator to allow the bars to set. This chilling procedure stiffens up the mixture, making it simpler to cut into individual bars without affecting structural integrity.

6. **Cut into bars:** Once the bars have fully set, remove the parchment paper to release the hardened mixture from the pan. Using a sharp knife, cut it into separate bars of your preferred size. The bars are now ready to be savored.

Nutritional Benefits: A Symphony of Nutrition

1. **Almonds contain plant-based protein and healthy fats:** Almonds offer plant-based protein, healthful monounsaturated fats, and important minerals. This combination increases satiety, cardiovascular health, and general well-being.

2. **Natural Sugars and Fiber in Dates:** Medjool dates have natural sugars that give energy as well as fiber, which assists digestion. The natural sweetness of dates makes these bars

delightful without the need for extra sweeteners.

3. **Sustained Energy from Rolled Oats:** Rolled oats deliver complex carbs and fiber, resulting in continual energy release. This makes almond and date energy bars a fantastic snack for keeping energy levels up throughout the day.

4. **Omega-3 Fatty Acids and Fiber from Chia Seeds:** add omega-3 fatty acids and extra fiber to the bars. These small seeds increase heart health, enhance satiety, and improve overall nutritional value.

5. **Creamy Texture and Nutrients of Almond Butter:** Almond butter provides a creamy smoothness to the bars while delivering healthy fats, protein, and vitamin E. It improves the nutty taste and aids in the bars' cohesiveness.

Chapter 7: Beverages for Optimal Eye Hydration

Green Tea Elixir with Citrus

1. **Green Tea Leaves and Bags:** At the center of this elixir is green tea, which is recognized for its many antioxidants and possible health perks. To achieve the greatest taste, use high-quality loose green tea leaves or bags.

2. **Fresh citrus (lemon, lime, or orange):** Citrus provides a tart edge to the elixir, making it more refreshing. Whether it's the acidic sharpness of lemon, the zing of lime, or the sweet scent of orange, citrus adds a dynamic layer of flavor.

3. **Fresh Mint Leaf (Optional):** Fresh mint leaves may add a herbal flavor and a layer of freshness to any cuisine. Mint balances the green tea and citrus, resulting in a lovely and pleasant mix.

4. **Honey or agave syrup (optional):** Use a tiny bit of honey or agave syrup to sweeten the elixir. This optional

additive enriches the overall taste without dominating the natural tastes of green tea and citrus.

Techniques:

1. **How to Brew Green Tea:** Start by brewing a cup of green tea with either loose leaves or tea bags. Allow the tea to steep for the appropriate period, generally 2-3 minutes, to extract the perfect balance of taste without bitterness.

2. **Add Fresh Citrus Zest:** While the green tea is still warm, peel and arrange fresh citrus in the cup. Whether you enjoy the vivid notes of lemon, the zesty sting of lime, or the fragrant flavor of orange, the zest fills the elixir with fresh vitality.

3. **Squeeze Citrus Juice:** After zesting, squeeze the juice of the citrus straight into the tea. Adjust the quantity to your satisfaction, balancing the acidity with the green tea's inherent sweetness.

4. **Add Mint Leaves (Optional):** To add a herbal taste, tear fresh mint leaves and blend them into the green tea elixir. The mint leaves enhance the scent and offer a refreshing aspect to the beverage.

5. **Optional:** Sweeten with honey or agave. To sweeten the elixir, sprinkle on some honey or agave syrup. Stir carefully to generate a uniform distribution of sweetness, keeping it modest so that the natural flavors may emerge. Serve over ice. Allow the green tea elixir to cool before pouring it over ice. This converts the elixir into a pleasant and hydrating beverage that is great for hot days or as a refreshing pick-me-up.

Nutritional Benefits:

1. **Antioxidants from green tea:** Green tea is abundant in antioxidants, notably catechins, which have been linked to a multitude of health advantages, including enhanced heart health and possible anti-inflammatory characteristics.

2. **Vitamin C from Citrus:** Citrus fruits, including lemon, lime, and orange, are rich in vitamin C. This vital vitamin boosts immunological function, skin health, and general well-being.

3. **Hydration and refreshment:** The mix of green tea and citrus gives a hydrating and refreshing experience. Staying hydrated boosts numerous biological systems and adds to overall vigor.

4. **Mint for Digestive Comfort:** If you add mint, it may aid with digestion. Its relaxing characteristics may help ease pain and create a feeling of well-being.

5. **Natural sweetness from honey or agave (optional):** The optional use of honey or agave syrup adds a hint of sweetness without the use of processed sweeteners. These natural sweeteners deliver gentle enjoyment.

Refreshing Cucumber and Mint Infused Water

Ingredients:

1. **Cucumber:** Cucumber, a hydrating and crisp ingredient, is key to this infused water. Cucumber not only has a wonderful flavor but also helps with hydration owing to its high water content.

2. **Fresh mint leaves:** Mint leaves deliver a rush of stimulating taste, changing simple water into a reviving elixir. Mint also has a subtle herbal aroma, which improves the overall freshness of the infused water.

3. **Fresh lime or lemon (optional):** Thin slices of fresh lemon or lime may give a zesty flavor. The zesty explosion improves the taste profile, resulting in a stunning blend of coolness and brightness.

4. **Ice cubes:** Ice cubes offer the final touch, ensuring that your cucumber- and mint-infused water is properly cold. The ice enriches the overall experience, particularly on warm days.

Techniques:

1. **Slicing cucumber:** Start by thoroughly cleaning the cucumber. Slice it thinly so that the pieces have a larger surface area to release their essence into the water more efficiently.

2. **Tearing Mint Leaves:** Tear fresh mint leaves to release the fragrant oils. This stage improves the absorption of minty freshness into the water, resulting in a lovely and revitalizing aroma.

3. **Optional:** Add citrus slices. If using citrus, finely slice a fresh lemon or lime. Orange slices not only offer a zesty flavor to the infused water, but they also make it more visually attractive.

4. **Assemble in a pitcher:** Place the cucumber slices, torn mint leaves, and citrus slices in a pitcher. Adjust the proportions to suit your taste, and don't be afraid to experiment with component ratios.

5. **Add ice cubes:** Fill the pitcher with ice cubes to ensure that the infused water is served cool. The ice cubes improve the overall freshness, making each sip delightful and joyful.

6. **Infusing and Chill:** Allow the ingredients to soak in the fridge for at least 1-2 hours, or overnight for a stronger taste. This chilling stage helps the cucumber, mint, and optional citrus fully blend with the water.

7. **Strain (optional):** Before serving, you may filter the infused water to remove the solid components or leave them for a visually pleasing presentation. Straining results in a smoother texture, especially if you prefer a clearer beverage.

Nutritional Benefits:

1. **Hydration with Cucumber:** Cucumber's high water content improves hydration and boosts general well-being. Staying hydrated is vital for a number of biological activities, from digestion to temperature control.

2. **Refreshing Aromatics of Mint:** Mint not only has a beautiful flavor, but it also includes components that may improve digestion and create a sensation of alertness.

3. **Citrus Vitamin Boost (Optional):** The inclusion of orange segments improves the infused water's vitamin C content. Vitamin C enhances immune health and provides a zesty tang to the taste.

4. **Chilled Satisfaction with Ice Cubes:** Ice cubes not only chill the infused water but also increase the overall enjoyment of each drink, particularly on hot days.

Carrot and Orange Juice Blend

Ingredients:

1. **Fresh carrots:** Fresh carrots, which are strong in beta-carotene and have a natural sweetness that complements the citrus flavors, serve as the foundation for this drink.

2. **Juicy oranges:** Juicy oranges add a blast of zesty brightness, delivering vitamin C and a lively taste that counteracts the earthiness of the carrots.

3. **Ginger (optional):** Fresh ginger may add spice and warmth to the meal. Ginger not only has a spicy taste but also has anti-inflammatory qualities.

Techniques:

1. **How to Prepare Carrots:** Begin by washing and peeling the carrots. Cut them into tiny pieces for easier juicing, eliminating any tough or woody regions.

2. **How to Peel and Segment Oranges:** Peel the oranges and cut them into pieces. This procedure guarantees that you obtain the beautiful richness of the oranges without the disagreeable pith.

3. **Optional ginger infusion:** If using ginger, peel a tiny amount and slice or grate it. This may be juiced with the carrots and oranges to offer a sense of spiciness.

4. **Juicing:** To extract the brilliant juice, process the carrots, oranges, and ginger (if included) in a high-quality juicer. Ensure that the final combination is smooth and well-integrated.

5. **Straining (optional):** To obtain a smoother juice, strain it over a fine mesh screen or cheesecloth to eliminate any pulp or fibrous remains. This stage is optional and dependent on personal choice.

6. **Chilling (optional):** Before serving, chill the juice in the refrigerator for a few minutes for a nice flavor. This increases the overall sharpness of the combination.

7. **Garnish (optional):** For a decorative touch, top the juice with an orange slice or a twist of orange peel. This not only provides visual attractiveness but also hints at the lovely citrus scent.

Nutritional Benefits:

1. **Carrots deliver a beta-carotene boost:** Carrots are abundant in beta-carotene, a precursor of vitamin A. This vitamin enhances eye health, skin brightness, and general immunological function.

2. **Vitamin C Infusion from Oranges:** Oranges feature a lot of vitamin C, a potent antioxidant that helps with immunity, collagen synthesis, and general health.

3. **Ginger's Anti-inflammatory Properties (Optional):** Ginger may have anti-inflammatory effects, aiding digestion and providing a slight warmth to the combination.

4. **Hydration and vital minerals:** The juice mix delivers hydration as well as vital minerals like potassium, which aid with electrolyte balance and general hydration.

Chapter 8: Meal Planning and Prep Tips

Creating Balanced and Eye-Boosting Menus

1. **Using colorful vegetables:** Begin by admiring the beauty of vibrant veggies. Carrots, bell peppers, spinach, and sweet potatoes contain antioxidants such as beta-carotene and lutein, which enhance eye health.

2. **Include Omega-3 Fatty Acids:** Include omega-3 fatty acids in your diet from foods such as fatty fish (salmon, mackerel), chia seeds, and flaxseed. These helpful lipids contribute to the structural integrity of the eye's retina.

3. **Going for Whole Grains:** Choose whole grains such as quinoa, brown rice, and oats to acquire complex carbs, fiber, and important elements. Whole grains

contribute to overall cardiovascular health, which promotes eye health.

4. **Embracing lean proteins:** Lean proteins, such as chicken, tofu, and lentils, are vital for the health of the eye muscles and tissues. Protein-rich diets boost the generation of enzymes important for visual function.

Creating A Balanced Menu

1. Breakfast:

Sunrise smoothie bowl: Start your day with a Sunrise Smoothie Bowl, which blends colorful berries, spinach, and a splash of omega-3-rich chia seeds. Top with almonds for extra crunch and vitamin E.

2. Mid-Morning Snack:

Greek Yogurt Parfait With Berries: Satisfy your mid-morning wants with a Greek yogurt parfait topped with antioxidant-rich berries and granola. The yogurt includes probiotics, which are important to general health.

3. Lunch:

Quinoa and Vegetable: Power Bowl Quinoa and Vegetable Power Bowl is a healthy lunch choice.

Combine bright greens, protein-packed chickpeas, and a drizzle of olive oil for a healthy fat boost.

4. **Afternoon pick-me-up:**

Trail Mix with Nuts and Dried Berries: Enjoy a handful of Trail Mix, which consists of nuts and dried fruit. This snack combines antioxidants, healthy fats, and energy-boosting nutrients.

5. **Dinner:**

Baked cod with lemon and herbs: Baked fish, seasoned with lemon and herbs, makes for a light but hearty meal. Cod is rich in omega-3 fatty acids, and the herbs give taste without adding too much salt.

6. **Evening Treat:**

Dark Chocolate and Berry Bliss Bites:

Enjoy a guilt-free evening treat with Dark Chocolate and Berry Bliss Bites. These nibbles blend the antioxidant benefits of dark chocolate with the enjoyment of mixed berries.

Key Principles

1. **Variety is visionary:** Diversify your diets to provide a wide variety of nutrients. Include a colorful array of

fruits and vegetables, nutritious grains, lean meats, and healthy fats.

2. **Portion Control:** Use purposeful portion control to maintain a healthy weight. Excess weight may induce illnesses such as diabetes, which may affect one's vision.

3. **Hydration Harmony:** Stay hydrated by eating a range of water-rich meals and drinking lots of water. Hydration helps general health, including ocular well-being.

4. **Limit processed indulgences:** Reduce your consumption of processed foods rich in refined sugars and harmful fats. Choose whole, nutrient-dense diets to boost overall health.

5. **Mindful Culinary Techniques:** Select cooking techniques that retain nutrients. Steaming, roasting, and grilling are ways to help foods maintain their nutritional value.

Smart Shopping for Eye-Healthy

Ingredients:

1.**Colorful Vegetables:** Fill your basket with a range of colorful vegetables, including kale, spinach, carrots, and bell peppers. These bright alternatives are rich in antioxidants like lutein and zeaxanthin, which are vital for sustaining eye health. Berries, such as blueberries and strawberries, add a pop of color. These berries have anthocyanins, which have anti-inflammatory and antioxidant qualities that are good for the eyes.

2. **Omega-3 Oasis:** Seek out fatty fish, such as salmon, mackerel, and trout. These fish contain high quantities of omega-3 fatty acids, notably DHA, which has been linked to better retinal function. Chia Seeds and Flaxseeds: Look in the bulk aisle for omega-3-rich seeds. Chia seeds and flaxseeds may be sprinkled over salads or mixed into smoothies for a plant-based dose of these vital fatty acids.

3. **Grain and Legume Enrichment:** Choose nutrient-dense whole grains such as quinoa. Quinoa, which is abundant in vitamins, minerals, and protein, supports overall wellbeing and helps with eye health. Fill your cart with legumes, such as lentils and chickpeas. These are good sources of plant-based protein, which increases the development of enzymes required to maintain eye health.

4. **Nut and Seed Haven: Almonds:** Grab a handful of almonds for a snack rich in vitamin E, an antioxidant

that protects the eyes from oxidative stress. Walnuts: Include walnuts on your shopping list for an omega-3 fatty acid and antioxidant boost, as well as a wonderful crunch to salads or yogurt.

Smart ways for eye-conscious shopping

1. **Read between the labels:** Prioritize complete, unprocessed foods. Fresh fruits, vegetables, and lean proteins are vital components of an eye-healthy diet. Beware of Added Sugars: Excess sugar intake has been linked to disorders such as diabetes, which can have an effect on eye health.

2. **Fresh and Seasonal Focus:** Prioritize Choose fresh, seasonal vegetables whenever they are available. Seasonal fruits and vegetables generally have increased nutritional qualities. Consider local and organic sources for vegetables. Because of the reduced travel time, locally obtained fresh foods may be more healthful.

3. **Diversify your cart:** Colorful Cart Diversity: Include a broad variety of colors in your cart. Different hues in fruits and vegetables suggest diverse antioxidants, giving complete eye care. Rotate protein sources to vary your nutritional intake. Alternating between fish, lean meats,

and plant-based proteins delivers a varied spectrum of necessary amino acids.

4. **Shopping List Prowess Plan Ahead**: Create a shopping list based on a balanced, eye-healthy diet plan. This guarantees that you cover all key nutrients while avoiding impulsive, less healthy choices. Stay informed about seasonal vegetables and integrate them into your shopping list. Seasonal foods are not only fresher, but they may also be less costly.

Simple Meal Prep Strategies for Busy Lifestyles

1. **Batch Cooking:** Begin by batch cooking proteins such as grilled chicken, roasted tofu, and lentils. These adaptable proteins may serve as the basis for a number of meals throughout the week. Batch-cook healthy grains like quinoa, brown rice, and farro. These grains may be used as the base for salads, bowls, or sides, offering a supply of complex carbs and fiber.

2. **Vegetable (Chop and store):** Spend time cutting a variety of veggies at once. Store them in containers or pre-portioned bags for quick access. Prepped vegetables

become ready-to-eat elements for stir-fries, salads, and omelets.

Choose to roast a significant number of veggies at the beginning of the week. Roasted vegetables may be simply added to wraps, grain bowls, or eaten as a savory side dish.

3. **Sauce and Dressing Mastery:** Create adaptable dressings and sauces that may be used in a number of cuisines. Consider adding a lemon vinaigrette, tahini sauce, or a fantastic pesto.

Marinades for Flavor: Make marinades for proteins during your prep period. Marinating ahead of time increases taste and saves on cooking time when it comes time for lunch.

4. **Strategic Storage Solution:** Portion Control: To make meal preparation simpler, invest in portion control containers. These containers not only aid with portion management, but they also make it easier to carry meals.

Freezer-Friendly Food

Use the freezer for storage. Soups, stews, and casseroles may be portioned and frozen for those busy days when cooking from scratch is a problem.

A Week of Efficiently Prepared Meals

1. **Breakfast:**

Overnight Oats with Mixed Berries: Prepare ahead of time by mixing oats, milk, and a little honey in jars. Add the mixed berries and soak them overnight. In the morning, grab a jar for a wholesome breakfast.

2. **Lunchtime:**

Quinoa Salad with Prepared Vegetables and Grilled Chicken:

Assemble and enjoy. Combine pre-cooked quinoa with prepped vegetables such as cherry tomatoes, cucumbers, and bell peppers. Add grilled chicken for a wonderful and well-balanced meal.

3. **Snack:**

Hummus with cut carrots and cucumber: Divide the hummus into containers and cut the carrots and cucumber. Keeping snack items on hand lessens hunger and adds fiber.

4. **Dinner Delight:**

One-Pan Roasted Vegetable and Tofu Bowl (Combine and Roast): Season prepared vegetables and tofu with your favorite seasonings before roasting on a sheet pan.

Serve over a bed of pre-cooked quinoa for a healthy and easy supper.

5. Sweet Finish:

Yogurt Parfait with Granola and Fresh Berries(Layer Ahead): Make yogurt parfaits by combining Greek yogurt, granola, and fresh berries. Preparing them in advance provides a pleasant and healthy dessert.

Key Principles

1. **Menu Diversity:** Create a menu with flexible foods that can be repeated for numerous meals. This lowers the need for extensive preparation sessions.

2. **Time-saving techniques:** Use a slow cooker, Instant Pot, or sheet pan meals. These gadgets expedite the cooking process.

3. **Flavor Flexibility:** Make adaptable components that can be readily adjusted with various spices or sauces. This keeps meals exciting without the need for substantial preparation.

4. **Prep Ritual:** Set aside a set day or time for meal preparation. Consistency creates efficiency, making meal preparation a tolerable and even joyful habit.

5. **Mindful Portioning:** Managing portion proportions during meal preparation ensures that meals are balanced and satisfying. It also streamlines the process of acquiring meals for individuals on the run.

Conclusion

Our investigation produces a tapestry of well-being in which every nutrient, meal, and culinary decision plays a vital part.

Let this understanding serve as a compass, directing us toward a future in which health is more than simply a destination but a constant, conscious journey. May the knowledge collected here serve as a source of inspiration, inspiring purposeful decisions that transcend the everyday and catapult our lives to new heights of living.

With each meal, drink, and nutritional activity, may we begin on a path of ongoing well-being, comprehending the fundamental link between our choices and the health we generate.

www.ingramcontent.com/pod-product-compliance
Lightning Source LLC
Chambersburg PA
CBHW061920270726
48658CB00005BB/1640